This book belongs to:

____

____

Personal Relaxation Inventory

Use the next few pages to determine how making relaxation an

everyday habit can change your life.

Why would you like to relax?

What could you accomplish?

Do you regularly take the time to relax?

When you do relax, does it come easily?

What steps will you take to become a more
relaxed person?

____
____
____
____
____
____
____
____
____
____
____
____

HERE BEGINS YOUR JOURNEY TO DAILY RELAXATION.

Week of:

How did you relax this week?

Writers choice: Take a hot bath.

Sunday

What did you do? ____

How did it feel?____

Monday

What did you do? ____

How did it feel?____

Tuesday

What did you do? ____

How did it feel?____

Wednesday

What did you do? ____

How did it feel?____

Thursday

What did you do? ____

How did it feel?____

Friday

What did you do? ____

How did it feel?____

Saturday

What did you do? ____

How did it feel?____

What did you like?

What would you change?

Week of:

How did you relax this week?

Writers choice: Practice yoga for 10 minutes.

Sunday

What did you do? ____

How did it feel?____

Monday

What did you do? ____

How did it feel?____

Tuesday

What did you do? ____

How did it feel?____

Wednesday

What did you do? ____

How did it feel?____

Thursday

What did you do? ____

How did it feel?____

Friday

What did you do? ____

How did it feel?____

Saturday

What did you do? ____

How did it feel?____

What did you like?

What would you change?

Week of:

How did you relax this week?

Writers choice: Mediation in the morning for 5 minutes.

Sunday

What did you do? ____

How did it feel?____

Monday

What did you do? ____

How did it feel?____

Tuesday

What did you do? ____

How did it feel?____

Wednesday

What did you do? ____

How did it feel?____

Thursday

What did you do? ____

How did it feel?____

Friday

What did you do? ____

How did it feel?____

Saturday

What did you do? ____

How did it feel?____

What did you like?

What would you change?

Week of:

How did you relax this week?

Writers choice: Listen to a mindfulness podcast.

Sunday

What did you do? _______________________________

How did it feel?_______________________________

Monday

What did you do? _______________________________

How did it feel?_______________________________

Tuesday

What did you do? _______________________________

How did it feel?_______________________________

Wednesday

What did you do? _______________________________

How did it feel?_______________________________

Thursday

What did you do? _______________________________

How did it feel?_______________________________

Friday

What did you do? _______________________________

How did it feel?_______________________________

Saturday

What did you do? _______________________________

How did it feel?_______________________________

What did you like?

What would you change?

Week of:

How did you relax this week?

Writers choice: Stretch for 5 minutes.

Sunday

What did you do? ____

How did it feel?____

Monday

What did you do? ____

How did it feel?____

Tuesday

What did you do? ____

How did it feel?____

Wednesday

What did you do? ____

How did it feel?____

Thursday

What did you do? ____

How did it feel?____

Friday

What did you do? ____

How did it feel?____

Saturday

What did you do? ____

How did it feel?____

What did you like?

What would you change?

Week of:

How did you relax this week?

Writers choice: Go on a walk.

Sunday

What did you do? ____

How did it feel?____

Monday

What did you do? ____

How did it feel?____

Tuesday

What did you do? ____

How did it feel?____

Wednesday

What did you do? ____

How did it feel?____

Thursday

What did you do? ____

How did it feel?____

Friday

What did you do? ____

How did it feel?____

Saturday

What did you do? ____

How did it feel?____

What did you like?

What would you change?

Week of:

How did you relax this week?

Writers choice: Take a hot bath.

Sunday

What did you do? ____

How did it feel?____

Monday

What did you do? ____

How did it feel?____

Tuesday

What did you do? ____

How did it feel?____

Wednesday

What did you do? ____

How did it feel?____

Thursday

What did you do? ____

How did it feel?____

Friday

What did you do? ____

How did it feel?____

Saturday

What did you do? ____

How did it feel?____

What did you like?

What would you change?

Week of:

How did you relax this week?

Writers choice: Watch your favorite movie.

Sunday

What did you do? ____

How did it feel?____

Monday

What did you do? ____

How did it feel?____

Tuesday

What did you do? ____

How did it feel?____

Wednesday

What did you do? ____

How did it feel?____

Thursday

What did you do? ____

How did it feel?____

Friday

What did you do? ____

How did it feel?____

Saturday

What did you do? ____

How did it feel?____

What did you like?

What would you change?

Week of:

How did you relax this week?

Writers choice: Read your favorite book.

Sunday

What did you do? _______________________________________

How did it feel?_______________________________________

Monday

What did you do? _______________________________________

How did it feel?_______________________________________

Tuesday

What did you do? _______________________________________

How did it feel?_______________________________________

Wednesday

What did you do? _______________________________________

How did it feel?_______________________________________

Thursday

What did you do? _______________________________________

How did it feel?_______________________________________

Friday

What did you do? _______________________________________

How did it feel?_______________________________________

Saturday

What did you do? _______________________________________

How did it feel?_______________________________________

What did you like?

What would you change?

Week of:

How did you relax this week?

Writers choice: Have a self-care spa day.

Sunday

What did you do? ____

How did it feel?____

Monday

What did you do? ____

How did it feel?____

Tuesday

What did you do? ____

How did it feel?____

Wednesday

What did you do? ____

How did it feel?____

Thursday

What did you do? ____

How did it feel?____

Friday

What did you do? ____

How did it feel?____

Saturday

What did you do? ____

How did it feel?____

What did you like?

What would you change?

Week of:

How did you relax this week?

Writers choice: Write!

Sunday

What did you do? ____

How did it feel?____

Monday

What did you do? ____

How did it feel?____

Tuesday

What did you do? ____

How did it feel?____

Wednesday

What did you do? ____

How did it feel?____

Thursday

What did you do? ____

How did it feel?____

Friday

What did you do? ____

How did it feel?____

Saturday

What did you do? ____

How did it feel?____

What did you like?

What would you change?

Week of:

How did you relax this week?

Writers choice: Call a dear friend.

Sunday

What did you do? ____

How did it feel?____

Monday

What did you do? ____

How did it feel?____

Tuesday

What did you do? ____

How did it feel?____

Wednesday

What did you do? ____

How did it feel?____

Thursday

What did you do? ____

How did it feel?____

Friday

What did you do? ____

How did it feel?____

Saturday

What did you do? ____

How did it feel?____

What did you like?

What would you change?

Week of:

How did you relax this week?

Writers choice: Practice breathing deeply.

Sunday

What did you do? ____

How did it feel?____

Monday

What did you do? ____

How did it feel?____

Tuesday

What did you do? ____

How did it feel?____

Wednesday

What did you do? ____

How did it feel?____

Thursday

What did you do? ____

How did it feel?____

Friday

What did you do? ____

How did it feel?____

Saturday

What did you do? ____

How did it feel?____

What did you like?

What would you change?

How did you relax this week?

Writers choice: Enjoy nature.

Sunday

What did you do? ____

How did it feel? ____

Monday

What did you do? ____

How did it feel? ____

Tuesday

What did you do? ____

How did it feel? ____

Wednesday

What did you do? ____

How did it feel? ____

Thursday

What did you do? ____

How did it feel? ____

Friday

What did you do? ____

How did it feel? ____

Saturday

What did you do? ____

How did it feel? ____

What did you like?

What would you change?

Week of:

How did you relax this week?

Writers choice: Listen to relaxing music.

Sunday

What did you do? ____

How did it feel?____

Monday

What did you do? ____

How did it feel?____

Tuesday

What did you do? ____

How did it feel?____

Wednesday

What did you do? ____

How did it feel?____

Thursday

What did you do? ____

How did it feel?____

Friday

What did you do? ____

How did it feel?____

Saturday

What did you do? ____

How did it feel?____

What did you like?

What would you change?

Week of:

How did you relax this week?

Writers choice: Get a massage.

Sunday

What did you do? ____

How did it feel?____

Monday

What did you do? ____

How did it feel?____

Tuesday

What did you do? ____

How did it feel?____

Wednesday

What did you do? ____

How did it feel?____

Thursday

What did you do? ____

How did it feel?____

Friday

What did you do? ____

How did it feel?____

Saturday

What did you do? ____

How did it feel?____

What did you like?

What would you change?

Week of:

How did you relax this week?

Writers choice: Go watch stand up comedy.

Sunday

What did you do? ____

How did it feel?____

Monday

What did you do? ____

How did it feel?____

Tuesday

What did you do? ____

How did it feel?____

Wednesday

What did you do? ____

How did it feel?____

Thursday

What did you do? ____

How did it feel?____

Friday

What did you do? ____

How did it feel?____

Saturday

What did you do? ____

How did it feel?____

What did you like?

What would you change?

Week of:

How did you relax this week?

Writers choice: Listen to guided imagery.

Sunday

What did you do? ____

How did it feel?____

Monday

What did you do? ____

How did it feel?____

Tuesday

What did you do? ____

How did it feel?____

Wednesday

What did you do? ____

How did it feel?____

Thursday

What did you do? ____

How did it feel?____

Friday

What did you do? ____

How did it feel?____

Saturday

What did you do? ____

How did it feel?____

What did you like?

What would you change?

How did you relax this week?

Writers choice: Go to an aquarium.

Sunday

What did you do? ____

How did it feel? ____

Monday

What did you do? ____

How did it feel? ____

Tuesday

What did you do? ____

How did it feel? ____

Wednesday

What did you do? ____

How did it feel? ____

Thursday

What did you do? ____

How did it feel? ____

Friday

What did you do? ____

How did it feel? ____

Saturday

What did you do? ____

How did it feel? ____

What did you like?

What would you change?

Week of:

How did you relax this week?

Writers choice: Light some candles.

Sunday

What did you do? ____

How did it feel?____

Monday

What did you do? ____

How did it feel?____

Tuesday

What did you do? ____

How did it feel?____

Wednesday

What did you do? ____

How did it feel?____

Thursday

What did you do? ____

How did it feel?____

Friday

What did you do? ____

How did it feel?____

Saturday

What did you do? ____

How did it feel?____

What did you like?

What would you change?

Week of:

How did you relax this week?

Writers choice: Bake a cake.

Sunday

What did you do? ____

How did it feel?____

Monday

What did you do? ____

How did it feel?____

Tuesday

What did you do? ____

How did it feel?____

Wednesday

What did you do? ____

How did it feel?____

Thursday

What did you do? ____

How did it feel?____

Friday

What did you do? ____

How did it feel?____

Saturday

What did you do? ____

How did it feel?____

What did you like?

What would you change?

Week of:

How did you relax this week?

Writers choice: Go flower shopping.

Sunday

What did you do? ______________________________________

How did it feel?______________________________________

Monday

What did you do? ______________________________________

How did it feel?______________________________________

Tuesday

What did you do? ______________________________________

How did it feel?______________________________________

Wednesday

What did you do? ______________________________________

How did it feel?______________________________________

Thursday

What did you do? ______________________________________

How did it feel?______________________________________

Friday

What did you do? ______________________________________

How did it feel?______________________________________

Saturday

What did you do? ______________________________________

How did it feel?______________________________________

What did you like?

What would you change?

Week of:

How did you relax this week?

Writers choice: Exercise.

Sunday

What did you do? ____

How did it feel?____

Monday

What did you do? ____

How did it feel?____

Tuesday

What did you do? ____

How did it feel?____

Wednesday

What did you do? ____

How did it feel?____

Thursday

What did you do? ____

How did it feel?____

Friday

What did you do? ____

How did it feel?____

Saturday

What did you do? ____

How did it feel?____

What did you like?

What would you change?

Week of:

How did you relax this week?

Writers choice: Take yourself out to dinner.

Sunday

What did you do? ____

How did it feel?____

Monday

What did you do? ____

How did it feel?____

Tuesday

What did you do? ____

How did it feel?____

Wednesday

What did you do? ____

How did it feel?____

Thursday

What did you do? ____

How did it feel?____

Friday

What did you do? ____

How did it feel?____

Saturday

What did you do? ____

How did it feel?____

What did you like?

What would you change?

Week of:

How did you relax this week?

Writers choice: Dance.

Sunday

What did you do? ____

How did it feel?____

Monday

What did you do? ____

How did it feel?____

Tuesday

What did you do? ____

How did it feel?____

Wednesday

What did you do? ____

How did it feel?____

Thursday

What did you do? ____

How did it feel?____

Friday

What did you do? ____

How did it feel?____

Saturday

What did you do? ____

How did it feel?____

What did you like?

What would you change?

Week of:

How did you relax this week?

Writers choice: Go on a hike.

Sunday

What did you do? ___________________________

How did it feel?___________________________

Monday

What did you do? ___________________________

How did it feel?___________________________

Tuesday

What did you do? ___________________________

How did it feel?___________________________

Wednesday

What did you do? ___________________________

How did it feel?___________________________

Thursday

What did you do? ___________________________

How did it feel?___________________________

Friday

What did you do? ___________________________

How did it feel?___________________________

Saturday

What did you do? ___________________________

How did it feel?___________________________

What did you like?

What would you change?

Week of:

How did you relax this week?

Writers choice: Go to the beach.

Sunday

What did you do? ____

How did it feel?____

Monday

What did you do? ____

How did it feel?____

Tuesday

What did you do? ____

How did it feel?____

Wednesday

What did you do? ____

How did it feel?____

Thursday

What did you do? ____

How did it feel?____

Friday

What did you do? ____

How did it feel?____

Saturday

What did you do? ____

How did it feel?____

What did you like?

What would you change?

Week of:

How did you relax this week?

Writers choice: Wear your coziest pjs.

Sunday

What did you do? ____

How did it feel?____

Monday

What did you do? ____

How did it feel?____

Tuesday

What did you do? ____

How did it feel?____

Wednesday

What did you do? ____

How did it feel?____

Thursday

What did you do? ____

How did it feel?____

Friday

What did you do? ____

How did it feel?____

Saturday

What did you do? ____

How did it feel?____

What did you like?

What would you change?

Week of:

How did you relax this week?

Writers choice: Play a board game with friends.

Sunday

What did you do? ____

How did it feel?____

Monday

What did you do? ____

How did it feel?____

Tuesday

What did you do? ____

How did it feel?____

Wednesday

What did you do? ____

How did it feel?____

Thursday

What did you do? ____

How did it feel?____

Friday

What did you do? ____

How did it feel?____

Saturday

What did you do? ____

How did it feel?____

What did you like?

What would you change?

Week of:

How did you relax this week?

Writers choice: Organize or clean (I promise this can work).

Sunday

What did you do? ____

How did it feel?____

Monday

What did you do? ____

How did it feel?____

Tuesday

What did you do? ____

How did it feel?____

Wednesday

What did you do? ____

How did it feel?____

Thursday

What did you do? ____

How did it feel?____

Friday

What did you do? ____

How did it feel?____

Saturday

What did you do? ____

How did it feel?____

What did you like?

What would you change?

Week of:

How did you relax this week?

Writers choice: Go to the movies.

Sunday

What did you do? ___________________________________

How did it feel?___________________________________

Monday

What did you do? ___________________________________

How did it feel?___________________________________

Tuesday

What did you do? ___________________________________

How did it feel?___________________________________

Wednesday

What did you do? ___________________________________

How did it feel?___________________________________

Thursday

What did you do? ___________________________________

How did it feel?___________________________________

Friday

What did you do? ___________________________________

How did it feel?___________________________________

Saturday

What did you do? ___________________________________

How did it feel?___________________________________

What did you like?

What would you change?

Week of:

How did you relax this week?

Writers choice: Walk your dog.

Sunday

What did you do? _______________________________________

How did it feel?_______________________________________

Monday

What did you do? _______________________________________

How did it feel?_______________________________________

Tuesday

What did you do? _______________________________________

How did it feel?_______________________________________

Wednesday

What did you do? _______________________________________

How did it feel?_______________________________________

Thursday

What did you do? _______________________________________

How did it feel?_______________________________________

Friday

What did you do? _______________________________________

How did it feel?_______________________________________

Saturday

What did you do? _______________________________________

How did it feel?_______________________________________

What did you like?

What would you change?

Week of:

How did you relax this week?

Writers choice: Pet your dog.

Sunday

What did you do? ____

How did it feel?____

Monday

What did you do? ____

How did it feel?____

Tuesday

What did you do? ____

How did it feel?____

Wednesday

What did you do? ____

How did it feel?____

Thursday

What did you do? ____

How did it feel?____

Friday

What did you do? ____

How did it feel?____

Saturday

What did you do? ____

How did it feel?____

What did you like?

What would you change?

Week of:

How did you relax this week?

Writers choice: Love your dog.

Sunday

What did you do? ____

How did it feel?____

Monday

What did you do? ____

How did it feel?____

Tuesday

What did you do? ____

How did it feel?____

Wednesday

What did you do? ____

How did it feel?____

Thursday

What did you do? ____

How did it feel?____

Friday

What did you do? ____

How did it feel?____

Saturday

What did you do? ____

How did it feel?____

What did you like?

What would you change?

Week of:

How did you relax this week?

Writers choice: Admire your cat from across the room.

Sunday

What did you do? ____

How did it feel?____

Monday

What did you do? ____

How did it feel?____

Tuesday

What did you do? ____

How did it feel?____

Wednesday

What did you do? ____

How did it feel?____

Thursday

What did you do? ____

How did it feel?____

Friday

What did you do? ____

How did it feel?____

Saturday

What did you do? ____

How did it feel?____

What did you like?

What would you change?

Week of:

How did you relax this week?

Writers choice: Create a gratitude journal.

Sunday

What did you do? ____

How did it feel?____

Monday

What did you do? ____

How did it feel?____

Tuesday

What did you do? ____

How did it feel?____

Wednesday

What did you do? ____

How did it feel?____

Thursday

What did you do? ____

How did it feel?____

Friday

What did you do? ____

How did it feel?____

Saturday

What did you do? ____

How did it feel?____

What did you like?

What would you change?

Week of:

How did you relax this week?

Writers choice: Spend quality time with the family.

Sunday

What did you do? ____

How did it feel?____

Monday

What did you do? ____

How did it feel?____

Tuesday

What did you do? ____

How did it feel?____

Wednesday

What did you do? ____

How did it feel?____

Thursday

What did you do? ____

How did it feel?____

Friday

What did you do? ____

How did it feel?____

Saturday

What did you do? ____

How did it feel?____

What did you like?

What would you change?

Week of:

How did you relax this week?

Writers choice: Eat your favorite meal.

Sunday

What did you do? ____

How did it feel?____

Monday

What did you do? ____

How did it feel?____

Tuesday

What did you do? ____

How did it feel?____

Wednesday

What did you do? ____

How did it feel?____

Thursday

What did you do? ____

How did it feel?____

Friday

What did you do? ____

How did it feel?____

Saturday

What did you do? ____

How did it feel?____

What did you like?

What would you change?

Week of:

How did you relax this week?

Writers choice: Sing at the top of your lungs.

Sunday

What did you do? ____

How did it feel?____

Monday

What did you do? ____

How did it feel?____

Tuesday

What did you do? ____

How did it feel?____

Wednesday

What did you do? ____

How did it feel?____

Thursday

What did you do? ____

How did it feel?____

Friday

What did you do? ____

How did it feel?____

Saturday

What did you do? ____

How did it feel?____

What did you like?

What would you change?

Week of:

How did you relax this week?

Writers choice: Sit in silence.

Sunday

What did you do? ____

How did it feel?____

Monday

What did you do? ____

How did it feel?____

Tuesday

What did you do? ____

How did it feel?____

Wednesday

What did you do? ____

How did it feel?____

Thursday

What did you do? ____

How did it feel?____

Friday

What did you do? ____

How did it feel?____

Saturday

What did you do? ____

How did it feel?____

What did you like?

What would you change?

Week of:

How did you relax this week?

Writers choice: Create a vision board.

Sunday

What did you do? ____

How did it feel?____

Monday

What did you do? ____

How did it feel?____

Tuesday

What did you do? ____

How did it feel?____

Wednesday

What did you do? ____

How did it feel?____

Thursday

What did you do? ____

How did it feel?____

Friday

What did you do? ____

How did it feel?____

Saturday

What did you do? ____

How did it feel?____

What did you like?

What would you change?

Week of:

How did you relax this week?

Writers choice: Enjoy a delicious dessert.

Sunday

What did you do? ____

How did it feel?____

Monday

What did you do? ____

How did it feel?____

Tuesday

What did you do? ____

How did it feel?____

Wednesday

What did you do? ____

How did it feel?____

Thursday

What did you do? ____

How did it feel?____

Friday

What did you do? ____

How did it feel?____

Saturday

What did you do? ____

How did it feel?____

What did you like?

What would you change?

Week of:

How did you relax this week?

Writers choice: Practice tai chi for 10 minutes.

Sunday

What did you do? ____

How did it feel?____

Monday

What did you do? ____

How did it feel?____

Tuesday

What did you do? ____

How did it feel?____

Wednesday

What did you do? ____

How did it feel?____

Thursday

What did you do? ____

How did it feel?____

Friday

What did you do? ____

How did it feel?____

Saturday

What did you do? ____

How did it feel?____

What did you like?

What would you change?

Week of:

How did you relax this week?

Writers choice: Use an adult coloring book.

Sunday

What did you do? ____

How did it feel?____

Monday

What did you do? ____

How did it feel?____

Tuesday

What did you do? ____

How did it feel?____

Wednesday

What did you do? ____

How did it feel?____

Thursday

What did you do? ____

How did it feel?____

Friday

What did you do? ____

How did it feel?____

Saturday

What did you do? ____

How did it feel?____

What did you like?

What would you change?

Week of:

How did you relax this week?

Writers choice: Scrapbook.

Sunday

What did you do? ____

How did it feel?____

Monday

What did you do? ____

How did it feel?____

Tuesday

What did you do? ____

How did it feel?____

Wednesday

What did you do? ____

How did it feel?____

Thursday

What did you do? ____

How did it feel?____

Friday

What did you do? ____

How did it feel?____

Saturday

What did you do? ____

How did it feel?____

What did you like?

What would you change?

Week of:

How did you relax this week?

Writers choice: Go on a picnic.

Sunday

What did you do? _____________________________________

How did it feel?_____________________________________

Monday

What did you do? _____________________________________

How did it feel?_____________________________________

Tuesday

What did you do? _____________________________________

How did it feel?_____________________________________

Wednesday

What did you do? _____________________________________

How did it feel?_____________________________________

Thursday

What did you do? _____________________________________

How did it feel?_____________________________________

Friday

What did you do? _____________________________________

How did it feel?_____________________________________

Saturday

What did you do? _____________________________________

How did it feel?_____________________________________

What did you like?

What would you change?

Week of:

How did you relax this week?

Writers choice: Watch the sunrise or sunset.

Sunday

What did you do? ____

How did it feel?____

Monday

What did you do? ____

How did it feel?____

Tuesday

What did you do? ____

How did it feel?____

Wednesday

What did you do? ____

How did it feel?____

Thursday

What did you do? ____

How did it feel?____

Friday

What did you do? ____

How did it feel?____

Saturday

What did you do? ____

How did it feel?____

What did you like?

What would you change?

Week of:

How did you relax this week?

Writers choice: Practice a new hobby.

Sunday

What did you do? ____

How did it feel?____

Monday

What did you do? ____

How did it feel?____

Tuesday

What did you do? ____

How did it feel?____

Wednesday

What did you do? ____

How did it feel?____

Thursday

What did you do? ____

How did it feel?____

Friday

What did you do? ____

How did it feel?____

Saturday

What did you do? ____

How did it feel?____

What did you like?

What would you change?

Week of:

How did you relax this week?

Writers choice: Doodle aimlessly.

Sunday

What did you do? ____

How did it feel?____

Monday

What did you do? ____

How did it feel?____

Tuesday

What did you do? ____

How did it feel?____

Wednesday

What did you do? ____

How did it feel?____

Thursday

What did you do? ____

How did it feel?____

Friday

What did you do? ____

How did it feel?____

Saturday

What did you do? ____

How did it feel?____

What did you like?

What would you change?

Week of:

How did you relax this week?

Writers choice: Give yourself a manicure.

Sunday

What did you do? ____

How did it feel?____

Monday

What did you do? ____

How did it feel?____

Tuesday

What did you do? ____

How did it feel?____

Wednesday

What did you do? ____

How did it feel?____

Thursday

What did you do? ____

How did it feel?____

Friday

What did you do? ____

How did it feel?____

Saturday

What did you do? ____

How did it feel?____

What did you like?

What would you change?

Week of:

How did you relax this week?

Writers choice: Do a crossword or sudoku.

Sunday

What did you do? ____

How did it feel?____

Monday

What did you do? ____

How did it feel?____

Tuesday

What did you do? ____

How did it feel?____

Wednesday

What did you do? ____

How did it feel?____

Thursday

What did you do? ____

How did it feel?____

Friday

What did you do? ____

How did it feel?____

Saturday

What did you do? ____

How did it feel?____

What did you like?

What would you change?

Week of:

How did you relax this week?

Do what works for you.

Sunday

What did you do? _______________________________________

How did it feel?_______________________________________

Monday

What did you do? _______________________________________

How did it feel?_______________________________________

Tuesday

What did you do? _______________________________________

How did it feel?_______________________________________

Wednesday

What did you do? _______________________________________

How did it feel?_______________________________________

Thursday

What did you do? _______________________________________

How did it feel?_______________________________________

Friday

What did you do? _______________________________________

How did it feel?_______________________________________

Saturday

What did you do? _______________________________________

How did it feel?_______________________________________

What did you like?

What would you change?

Personal Relaxation Inventory

Use the next few pages to determine how making relaxation an

everyday habit has changed your life.

Do you like to relax?

What have you accomplished through relaxation?

Do you regularly take the time to relax?

When you do relax, does it come easily?

Will you continue to take action to become a more relaxed person?

____
____
____
____
____
____
____
____
____
____
____
____
____
____

HERE ENDS YOUR JOURNEY TO DAILY RELAXATION.

Notes

Notes

Notes

Notes

Notes

Notes

Notes